The Joyful Path: A Guide to Eternal Happiness for Men and Women

PRAJASPRI DEO

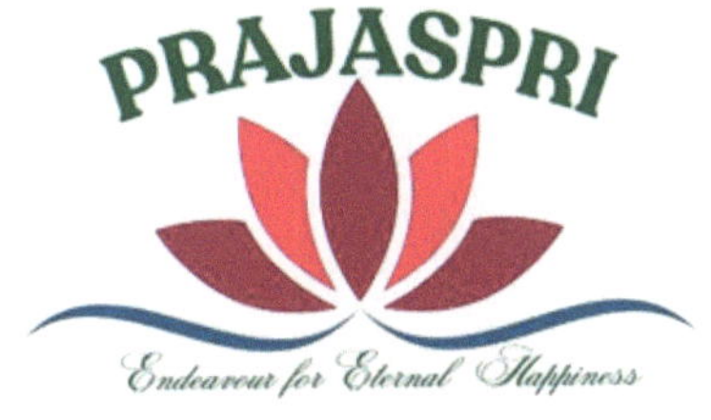

DEDICATION

"Dedicated to all those courageous souls embarking on the joyful path of self-discovery and inner transformation. May this guide illuminate your journey, inspiring you to embrace each moment with gratitude, kindness, and boundless joy. To the men and women who seek eternal happiness, may you find solace, guidance, and profound fulfillment along this luminous path.

CONTENTS

Upon the joyful path we tread,
In search of happiness, our daily bread.
Guided by light, both clear and bright,
Through trials and triumphs, day and night.

Men and women, hand in hand,
Exploring realms of joy so grand.
In each chapter, a lesson learned,
In every turn, new wisdom earned.

With courage firm and hearts ablaze,
We navigate life's winding maze.
Through laughter's dance and tear-stained eyes,
We find our bliss beneath the skies.

The Joyful Path, a cherished guide,
Leading us to joy that won't subside.
In its pages, truths untold,
For happiness is ours to behold.

So let us walk with spirits high,
Embracing life beneath the sky.
For on this path, together we roam,
Finding eternal happiness, our heart's true home.

CHAPTER ONE

ETERNAL HAPPINESS
BY DISCOVERING JOY
IN EVERY MOMENT

"Eternal Happiness by Discovering Joy in Every Moment" delves into the profound philosophy of finding enduring happiness within the fabric of daily existence. It invites introspection into the transformative power of embracing joy in the ordinary, fostering a mindset that transcends fleeting pleasures. This pursuit advocates for a shift in perspective, from seeking happiness in external circumstances to cultivating an inner reservoir of contentment. Through mindfulness and gratitude, it suggests that genuine and lasting happiness can be found in the present moment, amidst life's myriad experiences. This introspective journey promises not just fleeting moments of joy, but a sustainable path towards eternal happiness.

Understanding the concept of eternal happiness

Eternal happiness is a journey that many men and women embark upon in search of a fulfilling and joyous life. In "The Joyful Path: A Guide to Eternal Happiness for Men and Women", we delve into the various aspects of what it means to experience true and lasting happiness in every moment. Through mindfulness and meditation practices, individuals can find peace and contentment by being fully present in the here and now.

Cultivating gratitude and appreciation for the present moment is essential in the pursuit of eternal happiness. By acknowledging the blessings and beauty that surround us each day, we can learn to find joy in even the simplest of things. This practice of mindfulness allows us to let go of worries about the future or regrets from the past, and instead focus on the present moment where true happiness resides.

Finding happiness through self-discovery and personal growth is a transformative process that can lead to a more fulfilling life. By exploring our innermost thoughts, feelings, and desires, we can uncover our true purpose and passions, leading to a deeper sense of joy and fulfillment. Embracing simplicity and minimalism in our lives can also contribute to our overall happiness by freeing us from the burden of material possessions and allowing us to focus on what truly matters.

Nurturing relationships and connections with others is another key component of experiencing lasting joy and fulfillment. By fostering meaningful connections with loved ones and building strong bonds with friends and family, we can create a sense of belonging and support that enhances our overall well-being. Additionally, exploring the connection between physical health and emotional well-being can help us to achieve a more balanced and harmonious life.

Healing past traumas and releasing emotional baggage is necessary for creating a brighter future filled with happiness and contentment. By addressing unresolved issues from the past and letting go of negative emotions, we can make room for new experiences and opportunities for growth. Connecting with nature and the outdoors can also provide a sense of peace and harmony that can contribute to our overall sense of well-being. By incorporating spiritual practices and beliefs into our daily lives, we can find a deeper sense of purpose and fulfillment that transcends material desires and leads to a more meaningful and joyful existence.

Embracing the present moment for ultimate joy

In the pursuit of eternal happiness, it is essential to embrace the present moment with mindfulness and gratitude. The present moment is all we truly have, and by fully immersing ourselves in it, we can find ultimate joy and contentment. Never dwell on your past because you can't change it. By letting go of worries about the past or anxieties about the future, we can experience a sense of peace and fulfillment that transcends time.

Mindfulness and meditation practices are powerful tools for connecting with the present moment and cultivating a deep sense of inner peace. By slowing down and paying attention to our thoughts, emotions, and surroundings, we can find clarity and calm in the midst of life's chaos. Through regular mindfulness practice, we can train our minds to focus on the present moment, allowing us to let go of stress and worry and fully embrace the joy that is available to us in every moment.

Cultivating gratitude and appreciation for the present moment is another key to unlocking eternal happiness. By focusing on the blessings in our lives and expressing gratitude for the simple pleasures that surround us, we can shift our perspective from one of lack to one of abundance. When we take the time to acknowledge and appreciate the beauty and goodness that exists in the here and now, we open ourselves up to a deeper sense of joy and fulfillment.

Finding happiness through self-discovery and personal growth is a journey that begins with embracing the present moment. By exploring our true selves and uncovering our passions, values, and purpose, we can align our lives with what brings us the most joy and fulfillment. Through self-reflection and introspection, we can release limiting beliefs and fears that hold us back from experiencing true happiness, allowing us to step into our fullest potential and live a life of purpose and meaning.

Incorporating spiritual practices and beliefs into daily life is another way to deepen our connection with the present moment and find lasting joy and fulfillment. By nurturing our spiritual selves and connecting with something greater than ourselves, we can tap into a source of strength, peace, and wisdom that guides us on our journey towards eternal happiness. Whether through prayer, meditation, or simply connecting with nature, incorporating spiritual practices into our daily routine can help us find a deeper sense of purpose and meaning in our lives.

Cultivating a positive mindset for lasting happiness

Cultivating a positive mindset is essential for lasting happiness. In order to find joy in every moment, it is important to shift our focus towards positivity and gratitude. By adopting a positive mindset, we can train our minds to see the good in every situation, no matter how challenging it may be. This shift in perspective allows us to find happiness in even the smallest of moments, leading to a more fulfilling and joyful life.

Mindfulness and meditation practices are powerful tools for finding peace and contentment. By being present in the moment and quieting the mind through meditation, we can cultivate a sense of inner peace and tranquility. These practices help us to let go of negative thoughts and emotions, allowing us to experience a greater sense of happiness and fulfillment in our daily lives. By incorporating mindfulness and meditation into our daily routine, we can create a more positive and peaceful mindset that will lead to lasting happiness.

Cultivating gratitude and appreciation for the present moment is another key aspect of finding lasting joy. By focusing on the things we are grateful for, we can shift our perspective towards positivity and abundance. When we take the time to appreciate the beauty and blessings in our lives, we create a sense of fulfillment and contentment that can lead to lasting happiness. By practicing gratitude daily, we can train our minds to see the good in every situation and cultivate a positive mindset that will bring us joy in every moment.

Finding happiness through self-discovery and personal growth is a journey that requires us to look within ourselves and cultivate a deeper understanding of who we are. By exploring our passions, values, and beliefs, we can uncover our true purpose and create a life that aligns with our authentic selves. Through self-discovery and personal growth, we can cultivate a positive mindset that will lead to lasting happiness and fulfillment. By embracing simplicity and minimalism, we can create a more fulfilling life that is focused on the things that truly matter.

Nurturing relationships and connections is another key aspect of finding lasting joy and fulfillment. By surrounding ourselves with positive and supportive people, we can create a sense of community and belonging that enhances our overall well-being. By fostering deep and meaningful connections with others, we can cultivate a sense of happiness and fulfillment that will last a lifetime. By exploring the connection between physical health and emotional well-being, we can create a more balanced and harmonious life that promotes lasting happiness and fulfillment.

CHAPTER TWO

MINDFULNESS AND MEDITATION PRACTICES FOR FINDING PEACE AND CONTENTMENT

In the bustling chaos of modern life, the quest for inner peace and contentment has become paramount. "Mindfulness and Meditation Practices for Finding Peace and Contentment" offers a guiding light through this journey. Rooted in ancient wisdom yet tailored for contemporary living, this exploration illuminates the transformative potential of mindfulness and meditation. From focused breathing to mindful awareness, it unveils techniques to quiet the mind, anchor in the present, and cultivate a deep sense of tranquility. Through practical exercises and insightful guidance, this exploration serves as a roadmap for those seeking refuge from the storm, inviting a profound shift towards inner harmony and enduring contentment.

Introduction to mindfulness practices

In today's fast-paced world, many of us find ourselves constantly seeking happiness and fulfillment in external sources. We often overlook the power of mindfulness practices in helping us discover joy in every moment. This subchapter serves as an introduction to mindfulness practices for men and women who are on the path to eternal happiness. By incorporating these practices into our daily lives, we can cultivate peace and contentment within ourselves.

Mindfulness and meditation practices are powerful tools for finding peace and contentment in the present moment. By learning to quiet the mind and focus on the breath, we can create a sense of inner calm that transcends the chaos of everyday life. Through regular practice, we can train our minds to be more present and aware, allowing us to experience joy and fulfillment in even the simplest of moments.

Cultivating gratitude and appreciation for the present moment is another key aspect of mindfulness practices. By shifting our focus from what we lack to what we have, we can learn to find happiness in the here and now. This subchapter will explore techniques for developing a gratitude practice that can help us live more fully and joyfully.

Finding happiness through self-discovery and personal growth is a journey that requires mindfulness and introspection. By embracing simplicity and minimalism in our lives, we can create space for self-reflection and growth. This subchapter will provide guidance on how to let go of distractions and embrace a more fulfilling life through intentional living.

Nurturing relationships and connections are essential for lasting joy and fulfillment. Through mindfulness practices, we can learn to be more present and attentive in our interactions with others, fostering deeper connections and a greater sense of community. This subchapter will explore the importance of building meaningful relationships and how they contribute to our overall sense of happiness and well-being.

Benefits of meditation for emotional well-being

Meditation is a powerful tool for enhancing emotional well-being, offering numerous benefits for both men and women seeking eternal happiness. By incorporating mindfulness and meditation practices into daily life, individuals can find peace and contentment in every moment. Through the cultivation of gratitude and appreciation for the present moment, one can experience a greater sense of joy and fulfillment.

Finding happiness through self-discovery and personal growth is another key benefit of meditation. By embracing simplicity and minimalism, individuals can create a more fulfilling life free from unnecessary distractions. Nurturing relationships and connections with others is also essential for lasting joy and fulfillment, and meditation can help strengthen these bonds.

Exploring the connection between physical health and emotional well-being is crucial for overall happiness. By healing past traumas and releasing emotional baggage, individuals can create a brighter future filled with positivity and optimism. Connecting with nature and the outdoors can also provide a sense of peace and harmony, allowing for a deeper connection with oneself and the world around them.

Incorporating spiritual practices and beliefs into daily life can offer a deeper sense of purpose and fulfillment. By making meditation a regular part of one's routine, individuals can experience increased mental clarity, emotional stability, and a greater sense of inner peace. Ultimately, the benefits of meditation for emotional well-being are vast, offering a pathway to eternal happiness for all who seek it.

Techniques for incorporating mindfulness into daily life

Incorporating mindfulness into daily life is a powerful way to cultivate a sense of peace, contentment, and joy in every moment. By practicing mindfulness, we can learn to live more fully in the present, rather than getting caught up in worries about the future or regrets about the past. There are many techniques that can help us bring mindfulness into our daily routine, allowing us to experience the beauty and wonder of life in a more profound way.

One technique for incorporating mindfulness into daily life is to practice mindful breathing. By paying attention to our breath as we inhale and exhale, we can bring our awareness to the present moment and calm our minds. This simple practice can be done anywhere, at any time, and can help us to feel more grounded and centred in the midst of our busy lives.

Another technique for incorporating mindfulness into daily life is to practice mindful eating. By paying attention to the colours, textures, and flavours of our food, we can savour each bite and fully appreciate the nourishment it provides. This practice can help us to cultivate a sense of gratitude for the abundance in our lives and to develop a healthier relationship with food.

Incorporating mindfulness into daily life can also involve practicing mindful movement, such as yoga or tai chi. These practices can help us to connect with our bodies and with the present moment, allowing us to release tension and stress and to feel more at peace. By incorporating mindful movement into our daily routine, we can improve our physical health and emotional well-being, and experience a greater sense of vitality and joy.

Ultimately, the key to incorporating mindfulness into daily life is to approach each moment with an attitude of openness, curiosity, and compassion. By cultivating a mindful attitude, we can learn to appreciate the beauty and wonder of life in all its forms, and to find joy and fulfillment in every moment. By practicing mindfulness regularly, we can transform our lives and experience a deeper sense of peace, contentment, and happiness.

CHAPTER THREE

CULTIVATING GRATITUDE AND APPRECIATION FOR THE PRESENT MOMENT

"Cultivating Gratitude and Appreciation for the Present Moment" is a testament to the profound impact of mindfulness on our daily lives. In a world often consumed by the pursuit of the next milestone, this exploration champions the art of slowing down and savoring the here and now. Through deliberate practices and heartfelt reflection, it unveils the transformative power of gratitude in fostering resilience, enhancing well-being, and deepening connections with ourselves and others. From simple gestures to profound revelations, this journey celebrates the richness of each moment, inviting us to embrace life with open hearts and a renewed sense of appreciation for all that surrounds us.

The power of gratitude in finding joy

In the pursuit of eternal happiness, one of the most powerful tools we have at our disposal is gratitude. The act of expressing appreciation for the blessings in our lives can transform our mindset and bring about a sense of joy that is unmatched by any material possession. When we cultivate a spirit of gratitude, we open ourselves up to a world of abundance and possibility, allowing us to find joy in even the smallest of moments.

Practicing gratitude is not simply about saying thank you for the good things in our lives, but about truly feeling and embodying that sense of appreciation. It is about recognizing the beauty and wonder that surrounds us each day, from the warmth of the sun on our skin to the laughter of loved ones. By shifting our focus from what we lack to what we have, we can uncover a wellspring of joy that is always available to us, no matter our circumstances.

When we approach life with a mindset of gratitude, we begin to see the world through a different lens. Challenges and setbacks become opportunities for growth and learning, rather than obstacles to our happiness. We become more resilient in the face of adversity, knowing that even in the darkest moments, there is always something to be thankful for. Gratitude allows us to find joy in the present moment, regardless of what the future may hold.

Incorporating gratitude into our daily lives can be as simple as keeping a gratitude journal, where we write down three things we are thankful for each day. It can also involve expressing our appreciation to those around us, whether through a heartfelt thank you or a small act of kindness. By practicing gratitude regularly, we can rewire our brains to focus on the positive aspects of our lives, leading to a more joyful and fulfilling existence.

In the journey towards eternal happiness, cultivating gratitude is a powerful tool that can guide us towards a life filled with joy and contentment. By embracing the power of gratitude, we can find peace in every moment, connect more deeply with ourselves and others, and experience a sense of fulfillment that transcends our circumstances. Let us remember to be grateful for all that we have, and in doing so, discover a path to lasting happiness and joy.

Practicing appreciation for the simple things in life

In the hustle and bustle of modern life, it can be easy to get caught up in the never-ending cycle of striving for more. We are bombarded with messages that tell us we need to have the latest gadgets, the trendiest clothes, and the fanciest cars in order to be happy. But what if true happiness isn't found in material possessions, but in the simple things that are all around us?

Practicing appreciation for the simple things in life is a powerful way to shift our focus from what we lack to what we have. It allows us to fully experience the beauty of the present moment, whether it's the warmth of the sun on our skin, the sound of birds chirping in the morning, or the taste of a delicious meal shared with loved ones. By cultivating gratitude for these small moments, we can find joy in every aspect of our lives.

Mindfulness and meditation practices are essential tools for learning to appreciate the simple things in life. By quieting our minds and focusing on the present moment, we can fully immerse ourselves in the beauty of the world around us. These practices help us to let go of worries about the future or regrets about the past, allowing us to fully appreciate the richness of the present moment.

Cultivating gratitude and appreciation for the present moment is not just about feeling good in the moment – it has lasting effects on our overall well-being. Generally, people who practice gratitude regularly are happier, more optimistic, and have stronger immune systems. By taking the time to notice and appreciate the simple things in life, we can increase our overall sense of contentment and fulfillment.

Embracing simplicity and minimalism is another key aspect of finding joy in every moment. By decluttering our lives and focusing on what truly matters, we can create space for the things that bring us the most happiness. This could mean simplifying our schedules, letting go of toxic relationships, or spending more time in nature. By embracing simplicity, we can uncover the true treasures that life has to offer and find lasting joy and fulfillment.

Keeping a gratitude journal for daily reflection

Keeping a gratitude journal for daily reflection is a powerful tool that can help us cultivate a sense of appreciation for the present moment. In our fast-paced world, it's easy to get caught up in the hustle and bustle of daily life and forget to take a moment to reflect on the things we are thankful for. By keeping a gratitude journal, we can train our minds to focus on the positive aspects of our lives, which can lead to greater happiness and contentment.

Each day, take a few minutes to write down three things that you are grateful for. These can be big things, like a promotion at work or a beautiful sunset, or small things, like a warm cup of coffee or a friendly smile from a stranger. The key is to focus on the things that bring you joy and appreciation, no matter how big or small they may seem.

By regularly reflecting on the things we are grateful for, we can shift our mindset from one of lack and scarcity to one of abundance and gratitude. This shift in perspective can have a profound impact on our overall sense of well-being and happiness. Practicing gratitude can lead to increased feelings of positivity, improved relationships, and even better physical health.

In addition to writing down the things we are grateful for, it can also be helpful to reflect on why we are grateful for them. By delving deeper into the reasons behind our gratitude, we can gain a greater appreciation for the people, experiences, and things that bring us joy. This deeper level of reflection can help us cultivate a sense of mindfulness and presence in our daily lives.

Overall, keeping a gratitude journal for daily reflection is a simple yet powerful practice that can help us find joy in every moment. By taking the time to appreciate the good things in our lives, we can cultivate a sense of contentment and fulfillment that can lead to eternal happiness. So, grab a journal and start reflecting on the things you are grateful for – you may be surprised at how much joy it can bring to your life.

CHAPTER FOUR

FINDING HAPPINESS THROUGH SELF-DISCOVERY AND PERSONAL GROWTH

"Finding Happiness Through Self-Discovery and Personal Growth" embarks on a profound journey inward, illuminating the path towards enduring fulfillment. Rooted in the belief that true happiness resides within, this exploration champions the transformative process of self-discovery and continuous evolution. From unraveling limiting beliefs to nurturing strengths, it guides individuals towards a deeper understanding of themselves and their aspirations. Through introspection, self-awareness, and intentional growth, it unveils the keys to unlocking authentic happiness and living a purpose-driven life. This narrative serves as a beacon of inspiration for those seeking to navigate the complexities of existence with clarity, purpose, and unyielding joy.

Exploring your passions and purpose

Let us now delve into the importance of self-discovery and finding what truly brings joy and fulfillment into our lives. Being on the path to eternal happiness, it is crucial to understand that our passions and purpose play a significant role in shaping our overall well-being.

Many of us go through life without truly exploring our passions and purpose, leading to a sense of emptiness and lack of direction. By taking the time to immerse deep into what brings us joy and ignites our inner fire, we can uncover a sense of purpose that propels us forward on the path to eternal happiness.

Mindfulness and meditation practices can be powerful tools in helping us connect with our inner selves and uncovering our passions. By quieting the mind and listening to our inner voice, we can gain clarity on what truly brings us joy and fulfillment. Cultivating gratitude and appreciation for the present moment can also help us understand what truly matters to us and guide us towards our passions and purpose.

Finding happiness through self-discovery and personal growth is a journey that requires patience, dedication, and self-reflection. By embracing simplicity and minimalism in our lives, we can eliminate distractions and focus on what truly matters to us. Nurturing relationships and connections with others can also help us uncover our passions and purpose, as they often reflect back to us what we are truly passionate about.

Connecting with nature and the outdoors can provide us with a sense of peace and harmony, allowing us to connect with our inner selves and uncover our passions. By incorporating spiritual practices and beliefs into our daily lives, we can deepen our sense of purpose and fulfillment, guiding us towards eternal happiness. Ultimately, exploring our passions and purpose is a journey of self-discovery that can lead us to a more fulfilling and joyful life.

Overcoming self-limiting beliefs for personal growth

Overcoming self-limiting beliefs is a crucial step towards personal growth and achieving eternal happiness. Many of us hold onto negative beliefs about ourselves that can hinder our progress and prevent us from reaching our full potential. These beliefs may stem from past experiences, societal norms, or even our own insecurities. However, by recognizing and challenging these beliefs, we can break free from their limitations and pave the way for a more fulfilling life.

One of the first steps in overcoming self-limiting beliefs is to identify them. Take some time to reflect on the thoughts and beliefs that hold you back or cause you to doubt yourself. Are there patterns or recurring themes in your negative self-talk? Once you have identified these beliefs, you can begin to challenge them. Ask yourself if there is evidence to support these beliefs, or if they are simply holding you back out of fear or self-doubt.

Mindfulness and meditation practices can be powerful tools in overcoming self-limiting beliefs. By staying present in the moment and observing your thoughts without judgment, you can begin to untangle the web of negative beliefs that may be clouding your mind. Meditation can help you cultivate a sense of inner peace and clarity, allowing you to see yourself and your potential more clearly.

Cultivating gratitude and appreciation for the present moment is another key aspect of overcoming self-limiting beliefs. By focusing on the positive aspects of your life and acknowledging your strengths and accomplishments, you can shift your mindset from one of lack to one of abundance. Gratitude can help you see the potential for growth and happiness in every moment, even in the face of challenges or setbacks.

Finding happiness through self-discovery and personal growth is a journey that requires courage and commitment. It involves facing your fears, challenging your beliefs, and stepping outside of your comfort zone. However, the rewards of personal growth are immeasurable, leading to a deeper sense of fulfillment and lasting joy. By embracing simplicity, nurturing relationships, and connecting with nature, you can create a life filled with purpose, peace, and happiness. So, let go of your self-limiting beliefs and embark on the joyful path towards eternal happiness.

Setting goals for a fulfilling life

Setting goals for a fulfilling life is essential in order to live a life of joy and contentment. When we have clear goals in mind, we are able to focus our energy and efforts towards achieving them, leading to a sense of accomplishment and fulfillment. Let us explore the importance of setting goals that align with our values and desires, and how they can help us lead a more purposeful and meaningful life.

One of the first steps in setting goals for a fulfilling life is to take the time to reflect on what truly matters to us. This may involve exploring our values, passions, and dreams in order to identify what we want to achieve in life. By taking the time to clarify our goals, we can create a roadmap for our future that will guide us towards a more joyful and fulfilling existence.

Mindfulness and meditation practices can be powerful tools in helping us set and achieve our goals. By practicing mindfulness, we can cultivate a sense of clarity and focus that will enable us to better understand our desires and motivations. Meditation, on the other hand, can help us tap into our inner wisdom and intuition, guiding us towards goals that are in alignment with our true selves.

Cultivating gratitude and appreciation for the present moment is another important aspect of setting goals for a fulfilling life. When we are grateful for what we have and appreciate the beauty and abundance that surrounds us, we are able to approach our goals with a sense of positivity and optimism. Gratitude can also help us stay motivated and committed to our goals, even in the face of challenges and setbacks.

Finding happiness through self-discovery and personal growth is a key component of setting goals for a fulfilling life. When we take the time to explore our strengths, weaknesses, and beliefs, we can identify areas for growth and improvement that will help us achieve our goals. By embarking on a journey of self-discovery, we can uncover our true passions and desires, leading us towards a more fulfilling and joyful life.

Incorporating spiritual practices and beliefs into our daily lives can also help us set and achieve goals that are in alignment with our higher purpose. By connecting with our spiritual selves and tapping into a sense of divine guidance, we can gain clarity and insight into the goals that will bring us the most joy and fulfillment. By setting goals that are in alignment with our spiritual beliefs and values, we can create a life that is truly fulfilling and meaningful.

CHAPTER FIVE

EMBRACING SIMPLICITY AND MINIMALISM FOR A MORE FULFILLING LIFE

"Embracing Simplicity and Minimalism for a More Fulfilling Life" advocates for a paradigm shift in the pursuit of happiness. Amidst the clamor of consumerism and excess, this exploration champions the liberating ethos of minimalism. It extols the virtues of decluttering not just physical possessions, but also mental clutter, to uncover what truly matters. By embracing simplicity, it invites a deeper connection to oneself and the world, fostering mindfulness and gratitude. Through intentional living and conscious consumption, this narrative offers a roadmap to liberation from the trappings of materialism, leading to a more meaningful and fulfilling existence.

Decluttering your physical and mental space

In the journey towards eternal happiness, it is essential to declutter both our physical and mental spaces. Clutter can weigh us down, both physically and mentally, and prevent us from experiencing true joy and contentment in our lives. By clearing out the unnecessary and focusing on what truly matters, we can create a sense of peace and harmony within ourselves.

Physical decluttering involves getting rid of material possessions that no longer serve a purpose or bring us joy. This could mean clearing out our closets, getting rid of old paperwork, or simplifying our living spaces. By letting go of excess belongings, we create room for new energy and opportunities to flow into our lives.

Similarly, mental decluttering involves letting go of negative thoughts, limiting beliefs, and emotional baggage that may be holding us back. This could involve practicing mindfulness and meditation to quiet the mind and focus on the present moment. By releasing mental clutter, we can create space for positivity, gratitude, and joy to flourish.

Embracing simplicity and minimalism is key to living a more fulfilling life.

By focusing on what truly matters and letting go of the rest, we can cultivate a sense of peace and contentment within ourselves. This could mean simplifying our daily routines, decluttering our schedules, and prioritizing self-care and self-discovery.

By decluttering our physical and mental spaces, we can create a more joyful and fulfilling life for ourselves. Through mindfulness, gratitude, and simplicity, we can find peace and contentment in every moment. By letting go of what no longer serves us and focusing on what truly matters, we can discover eternal happiness within ourselves.

Living a minimalist lifestyle for inner peace

Living a minimalist lifestyle is a powerful way to cultivate inner peace and find lasting happiness. In today's fast-paced world filled with consumerism and materialism, it can be easy to get caught up in the cycle of wanting more and more. The quest to achieve more never ends. However, by embracing simplicity and minimalism, we can free ourselves from the burden of excess and focus on what truly matters.

Minimalism is not just about decluttering our physical space, but also decluttering our minds and hearts. By letting go of unnecessary possessions, commitments, and distractions, we create space for peace, clarity, and contentment to enter our lives. This can lead to a greater sense of freedom and fulfillment, as we learn to appreciate and savour the present moment.

One of the key benefits of living a minimalist lifestyle is the reduction of stress and anxiety. When we are constantly surrounded by clutter and chaos, it can be difficult to find peace and relaxation. By simplifying our surroundings and our lives, we can create a sense of calm and tranquillity that allows us to better cope with the challenges and uncertainties of life.

In addition to reducing stress, minimalism can also help us cultivate gratitude and appreciation for the present moment. When we are not constantly chasing after more possessions or achievements, we can learn to be content with what we have and find joy in the simple pleasures of life. This shift in mindset can lead to a greater sense of fulfillment and happiness, as we learn to find beauty and wonder in the everyday moments.

Ultimately, living a minimalist lifestyle is about prioritizing what truly matters to us and letting go of the rest. By simplifying our lives, we can create space for inner peace, joy, and contentment to flourish. Whether it's decluttering our physical space, simplifying our schedules, or letting go of toxic relationships, embracing minimalism can lead to a more fulfilling and meaningful life.

Simplifying your daily routines for increased happiness

In our fast-paced and hectic world, it can be easy to get caught up in the daily grind and forget to take care of ourselves. However, simplifying our daily routines can lead to increased happiness and overall well-being. By streamlining our tasks and focusing on what truly matters, we can find more joy in every moment.

One way to simplify your daily routine is to prioritize your tasks and eliminate any unnecessary activities. By focusing on what is truly important to you, you can reduce stress and create more time for activities that bring you happiness. This could mean cutting out time-wasting activities or delegating tasks to others to free up your schedule.

Another way to simplify your daily routine is to practice mindfulness and meditation. These practices can help you stay present in the moment and reduce anxiety and stress. By taking a few moments each day to centre yourself and quiet your mind, you can cultivate a sense of peace and contentment that will carry you through the day.

Cultivating gratitude and appreciation for the present moment is another key to simplifying your daily routine and finding happiness. By focusing on the positive aspects of your life and practicing gratitude for the little things, you can shift your mindset towards joy and fulfillment. This can lead to a more positive outlook on life and a greater sense of overall well-being.

Finding happiness through self-discovery and personal growth is also essential for simplifying your daily routine. By taking the time to explore your interests, values, and passions, you can align your daily activities with what truly brings you joy. This can lead to a more fulfilling life and a greater sense of purpose and satisfaction. By embracing simplicity and minimalism in your daily routines, you can create a more peaceful and harmonious environment for yourself. Removing clutter and excess possessions can free up mental space and create a sense of calm in your life. This can lead to increased happiness and contentment as you focus on what truly matters to you.

CHAPTER SIX

NURTURING RELATIONSHIPS AND CONNECTIONS FOR LASTING JOY AND FULFILLMENT

"Nurturing Relationships and Connections for Lasting Joy and Fulfillment" embarks on an exploration of the profound impact of human connection on our well-being. Beyond material pursuits, this journey delves into the heart of what truly enriches our lives: meaningful relationships. It celebrates the power of authentic connections, emphasizing empathy, communication, and mutual support as pillars of enduring joy. Through acts of kindness, understanding, and shared experiences, this narrative unveils the transformative potential of cultivating and nurturing relationships. It serves as a guiding light, reminding us that the true essence of fulfillment lies not in solitude, but in the warmth and depth of genuine human connection.

Building meaningful connections with others

Building meaningful connections with others is an essential aspect of finding joy and fulfillment in life. As social beings, humans thrive on the connections we make with others, whether they be friends, family, colleagues, or even strangers. These connections can bring a sense of belonging, support, and love that enrich our lives in ways that nothing else can.

To build meaningful connections with others, it is important to first be open and vulnerable. Authenticity is key in forming genuine relationships that are built on trust and mutual respect. By being honest and true to yourself, you invite others to do the same, creating a bond that is deep and lasting.

Listening is another crucial component of building meaningful connections. Taking the time to truly listen to others, to understand their thoughts, feelings, and experiences, shows that you value and care for them. This act of empathy and compassion fosters a sense of connection that goes beyond surface-level interactions.

In our fast-paced, digitally-driven world, it can be easy to overlook the importance of face-to-face interactions. However, nothing can replace the power of human connection that comes from being physically present with another person. Making time for meaningful conversations, shared experiences, and quality time spent together can deepen your relationships and bring immense joy and fulfillment.

Ultimately, building meaningful connections with others is a practice that requires time, effort, and intention. By nurturing these relationships and investing in the people around you, you not only enhance your own sense of happiness and well-being but also contribute to a more connected and compassionate world. Embrace the joy that comes from building meaningful connections with others, and watch as your life becomes richer and more fulfilling in every way.

Communicating effectively in relationships

In any relationship, communication is key. It is the foundation upon which trust, understanding, and connection are built. Without effective communication, misunderstandings can arise, feelings can be hurt, and relationships can suffer. Therefore, it is crucial for both men and women to learn how to communicate effectively in their relationships in order to foster joy and fulfillment.

One of the most important aspects of effective communication in relationships is active listening. This means truly being present and engaged in the conversation, listening not just to respond but to understand. When we listen actively, we show our partner that we value their thoughts and feelings, which can strengthen the bond between us.

Another important factor in effective communication is expressing ourselves honestly and openly. It is important to communicate our needs, desires, and concerns in a clear and respectful manner. By being honest and vulnerable with our partners, we create a safe space for open and honest communication to flourish.

In addition to active listening and honest expression, it is also important to practice empathy and compassion in our communication. This means trying to see things from our partner's perspective, showing understanding and empathy for their feelings, and responding with kindness and compassion. By practicing empathy, we can create deeper connections and foster greater understanding in our relationships.

Overall, effective communication in relationships is a skill that can be cultivated and improved over time. By practicing active listening, honest expression, empathy, and compassion, men and women can strengthen their relationships, deepen their connections, and experience greater joy and fulfillment in their lives.

Finding joy in giving back to your community

In the journey towards eternal happiness, one of the most powerful ways to experience joy is by giving back to your community. When we contribute to the well-being of others, we not only make a positive impact on the world around us, but we also cultivate a deep sense of fulfillment within ourselves. Whether it's volunteering at a local charity, donating to a cause you care about, or simply lending a helping hand to a neighbour in need, the act of giving back is a surefire way to elevate your spirits and find joy in every moment.

Mindfulness and meditation practices can greatly enhance the experience of giving back to your community. By being fully present and aware of your actions, you can approach your acts of kindness with intention and sincerity. Take the time to reflect on the impact you are making and the gratitude you feel for the opportunity to contribute in a meaningful way. Through mindfulness, you can cultivate a deeper connection to your community and a greater sense of joy in your giving.

Cultivating gratitude and appreciation for the present moment is essential when it comes to finding joy in giving back. When we focus on the positive aspects of our lives and the blessings we have, we naturally become more inclined to share our abundance with others. By expressing gratitude for the opportunities to give back and the impact it has on both ourselves and those we help, we can amplify the joy we experience and create a ripple effect of positivity in our community.

Finding happiness through self-discovery and personal growth is intricately linked to the act of giving back to your community. As you explore your values, passions, and strengths, you can identify unique ways to contribute to the world around you. By aligning your actions with your authentic self, you can experience a deep sense of fulfillment and purpose in your giving. Embrace the opportunity to grow and evolve through your acts of kindness, and watch as your joy expands exponentially.

Embracing simplicity and minimalism can also play a key role in finding joy in giving back to your community. By decluttering your life and focusing on what truly matters, you can create more space for generosity and compassion. Simplify your lifestyle to make room for meaningful connections and opportunities to give back, and you will find that the joy you experience is not only profound but also sustainable. Remember, the path to eternal happiness is paved with acts of kindness and selflessness – so embrace the joy of giving back to your community and watch as your life becomes infinitely more fulfilling.

CHAPTER SEVEN

EXPLORING THE CONNECTION BETWEEN PHYSICAL HEALTH AND EMOTIONAL WELL-BEING

"Exploring the Connection Between Physical Health and Emotional Well-Being" delves into the intricate relationship between our bodies and minds. This exploration unveils how our physical health profoundly impacts our emotional well-being, and vice versa. From the chemical reactions triggered by exercise to the psychological effects of chronic stress, every aspect of our health intertwines to shape our overall wellness. Through scientific insights and practical strategies, this narrative navigates the synergistic dance between physical vitality and emotional resilience. It advocates for holistic self-care practices that honor the interconnectedness of our physical and emotional selves, fostering a balanced and thriving existence.

The impact of exercise on mental health

Exercise has long been hailed for its physical benefits, but its impact on mental health is equally profound. Regular physical activity has been shown to reduce symptoms of anxiety and depression, improve mood, and enhance overall well-being. In fact, studies have found that exercise can be just as effective as medication in treating mild to moderate depression. For men and women seeking eternal happiness, incorporating exercise into their daily routine can be a powerful tool in maintaining mental health.

One of the key ways in which exercise benefits mental health is through the release of endorphins, often referred to as the "feel-good" hormones. When we engage in physical activity, our bodies produce these chemicals, which help to reduce feelings of stress and anxiety while promoting a sense of relaxation and well-being. This natural high can be a powerful mood booster, making exercise a valuable tool for those looking to cultivate joy in every moment.

Furthermore, exercise has been shown to improve cognitive function and enhance mental clarity. Physical activity increases blood flow to the brain, which can help to sharpen focus, improve memory, and boost overall cognitive function. For people looking to find peace and contentment through mindfulness and meditation practices, incorporating exercise into their routine can help to support mental clarity and enhance their ability to stay present in the moment.

In addition to its immediate mood-boosting effects, exercise can also have long-term benefits for mental health. Regular physical activity has been linked to a reduced risk of developing depression and anxiety disorders, as well as a lower likelihood of experiencing cognitive decline with age. By cultivating gratitude and appreciation for the present moment through exercise, men and women can set themselves up for a lifetime of mental well-being and fulfillment.

Incorporating exercise into your daily routine is a simple yet powerful way to support your mental health and well-being. Whether you prefer to go for a run, take a yoga class, or simply go for a walk-in nature, finding ways to stay active can have a profound impact on your overall happiness and contentment. By embracing simplicity and minimalism in your approach to exercise, you can create a sustainable routine that supports your mental health for years to come.

Eating for emotional well-being

In the journey towards eternal happiness, it is essential to recognize the important role that our diet plays in our emotional well-being. What we eat not only affects our physical health but also has a direct impact on our mood, energy levels, and overall outlook on life. By making conscious choices about what we put into our bodies, we can cultivate a sense of balance and harmony that contributes to our emotional well-being.

When it comes to eating for emotional well-being, it is important to focus on nourishing our bodies with whole, nutrient-rich foods. This means incorporating plenty of fruits, vegetables, whole grains, lean proteins, and healthy fats into our diet. These foods provide essential vitamins, minerals, and antioxidants that support our mental health and help regulate our mood. By avoiding processed foods, sugary snacks, and excessive caffeine, we can prevent mood swings, energy crashes, and feelings of irritability.

Mindful eating is another important aspect of eating for emotional well-being. By paying attention to the colours, textures, and flavours of our food, we can fully savour the experience of eating and connect with our bodies on a deeper level. This practice not only helps us make healthier food choices but also allows us to appreciate the nourishment and pleasure that food can bring. By slowing down and savouring each bite, we can cultivate a sense of gratitude and mindfulness that enhances our overall well-being.

Incorporating self-care practices into our daily routine can also support our emotional well-being. Taking the time to prepare and enjoy nourishing meals can be a form of self-love and self-care that boosts our mood and nurtures our soul. By setting aside time to cook, eat, and savour our meals, we can create a sense of peace and contentment that carries over into other areas of our lives. Eating mindfully and with intention can be a powerful form of self-care that nourishes our body, mind, and spirit.

In conclusion, eating for emotional well-being is an essential component of the path to eternal happiness. By choosing whole, nutrient-rich foods, practicing mindful eating, and incorporating self-care practices into our daily routine, we can support our emotional health and cultivate a sense of balance and harmony. By nourishing our bodies with love and intention, we can create a foundation of well-being that allows us to experience joy and fulfillment in every moment.

Practicing self-care for a balanced life

In the journey towards eternal happiness, practicing self-care is essential for maintaining a balanced life. It is important for both men and women to prioritize their own well-being in order to experience true joy in every moment. Self-care encompasses various aspects of our lives, including physical, emotional, mental, and spiritual well-being. By taking care of ourselves on all levels, we can cultivate a sense of peace and contentment that will lead to a more fulfilling life.

One way to practice self-care is through mindfulness and meditation practices. By taking time to quiet the mind and focus on the present moment, we can find inner peace and clarity. Mindfulness allows us to become more aware of our thoughts and emotions, helping us to release negative patterns and cultivate a sense of gratitude and appreciation for the present moment. Through meditation, we can connect with our inner selves and tap into a source of deep inner peace that will guide us towards happiness and fulfillment.

Cultivating gratitude and appreciation for the present moment is another important aspect of self-care. By focusing on the positive aspects of our lives and expressing gratitude for the blessings we have, we can shift our perspective to one of abundance and joy. Gratitude has the power to transform our outlook on life and help us to find happiness in even the smallest moments. By practicing gratitude daily, we can create a more positive and fulfilling life for ourselves and those around us.

Finding happiness through self-discovery and personal growth is a journey that requires self-care and self-reflection. By exploring our passions, values, and beliefs, we can uncover our true selves and align our lives with our authentic desires. Personal growth allows us to break free from limiting beliefs and step into our full potential, leading to a deeper sense of fulfillment and purpose. By embracing self-discovery as a form of self-care, we can create a life that is rich in meaning and joy.

Embracing simplicity and minimalism is another way to practice self-care and create a more fulfilling life. By decluttering our physical space and simplifying our lives, we can reduce stress and overwhelm, allowing us to focus on what truly matters. Minimalism encourages us to let go of material possessions and external pressures, and instead, prioritize our inner well-being and relationships. By embracing simplicity, we can create a sense of calm and clarity that will lead to lasting joy and fulfillment in our lives.

CHAPTER EIGHT

HEALING PAST TRAUMAS AND RELEASING EMOTIONAL BAGGAGE FOR A BRIGHTER FUTURE

"Healing Past Traumas and Releasing Emotional Baggage for a Brighter Future" embarks on a profound journey of self-discovery and liberation. This exploration delves into the transformative power of confronting and processing past traumas, freeing ourselves from the chains of emotional burden. Through introspection, therapeutic techniques, and resilience-building strategies, it unveils a path towards healing and renewal. By acknowledging our wounds with courage and compassion, we reclaim agency over our narratives, paving the way for a brighter, more empowered future. This narrative serves as a beacon of hope, illuminating the transformative potential of embracing our scars and stepping into the light of wholeness.

Understanding the effects of past traumas on your present happiness

Understanding the effects of past traumas on your present happiness is a crucial step towards achieving eternal joy. Many of us carry emotional baggage from our past experiences, whether it be childhood traumas, toxic relationships, or painful memories. These unresolved issues can manifest in various ways, impacting our mental health and overall well-being. By acknowledging and addressing these past traumas, we can begin the healing process and pave the way for a brighter future filled with happiness and fulfillment.

It is important to recognize that past traumas have a significant impact on our present happiness. When we suppress or ignore these painful experiences, they can continue to haunt us, affecting our relationships, self-esteem, and overall quality of life. By facing our past traumas head-on, we can begin to release the emotional baggage that has been weighing us down and holding us back from experiencing true joy and contentment in the present moment.

Healing past traumas requires courage, self-reflection, and a willingness to confront the pain that we have been avoiding. This process may involve seeking therapy, practicing mindfulness and meditation, or engaging in other forms of self-care and self-discovery. By taking the time to explore and process our past traumas, we can begin to release the negative emotions associated with these experiences and create space for healing, growth, and transformation.

By cultivating gratitude and appreciation for the present moment, we can learn to let go of the past and embrace the beauty and joy that surround us. By focusing on the blessings and abundance in our lives, we can shift our perspective from one of lack and suffering to one of gratitude and fulfillment. This shift in mindset can help us to release the grip of past traumas and open ourselves up to a brighter future filled with happiness, peace, and contentment.

Incorporating spiritual practices and beliefs into our daily lives can also help us to heal past traumas and find a deeper sense of purpose and fulfillment. By connecting with our higher selves, the universe, or a higher power, we can tap into a source of strength, guidance, and love that can support us on our journey towards healing and happiness. By integrating spirituality into our daily routines, we can cultivate a sense of peace, harmony, and connection that can help us to release past traumas and embrace a brighter future filled with eternal joy.

Techniques for processing and healing emotional wounds

Emotional wounds are a natural part of the human experience, but they can often be difficult to process and heal. In "The Joyful Path: A Guide to Eternal Happiness for Men and Women," we explore various techniques for addressing these wounds and finding peace and contentment in every moment. By understanding the root causes of our emotional pain and learning how to release it, we can open ourselves up to a brighter future full of joy and fulfillment.

One powerful technique for processing and healing emotional wounds is mindfulness and meditation practices. By bringing our awareness to the present moment and learning to observe our thoughts and feelings without judgment, we can begin to unravel the layers of emotional baggage that have been weighing us down. Through regular meditation practice, we can cultivate a sense of inner peace and contentment that allows us to let go of past traumas and embrace a more joyful way of being.

Cultivating gratitude and appreciation for the present moment is another essential tool for healing emotional wounds. By focusing on the positive aspects of our lives and expressing gratitude for the blessings we have, we can shift our perspective from one of lack and suffering to one of abundance and joy. This practice of gratitude can help us to release negative emotions and cultivate a sense of inner peace and contentment that is essential for true happiness.

Finding happiness through self-discovery and personal growth is also key to healing emotional wounds. By exploring our innermost thoughts and feelings, we can begin to uncover the root causes of our emotional pain and work towards healing and transformation. Through practices such as journaling, therapy, and self-reflection, we can gain a deeper understanding of ourselves and our emotional wounds, allowing us to release them and move forward with a renewed sense of purpose and fulfillment.

Incorporating spiritual practices and beliefs into daily life can also be a powerful tool for healing emotional wounds. By connecting with a higher power or spiritual source, we can gain a sense of perspective and purpose that can help us to navigate life's challenges with grace and resilience. Whether through prayer, meditation, or other spiritual practices, fostering a deeper connection to something greater than ourselves can provide comfort and healing in times of emotional distress.

Forgiveness as a path to inner peace

Forgiveness is a powerful tool that can lead us on the path to inner peace. When we hold onto grudges and resentment, we carry a heavy burden that weighs us down and prevents us from experiencing true happiness. By choosing to forgive those who have wronged us, we free ourselves from the chains of anger and bitterness, allowing space for love and compassion to flourish in our hearts. "To err is human, but to forgive is divine".

In the journey towards eternal happiness, forgiveness plays a crucial role in our mental and emotional well-being. Holding onto past hurts only serves to keep us stuck in a cycle of pain and suffering. When we choose to forgive, we release ourselves from the grip of negative emotions and open ourselves up to a world of possibilities and opportunities for growth and healing.

Mindfulness and meditation practices can help us cultivate the mindset needed to forgive and let go of past grievances. By staying present in the moment and observing our thoughts and emotions without judgment, we can gain a deeper understanding of our inner workings and find the strength to forgive ourselves and others. Through regular meditation practice, we can learn to cultivate a sense of inner peace and contentment that transcends any external circumstances.

Forgiveness is not always easy, especially when the wounds run deep. However, by choosing to forgive, we empower ourselves to break free from the chains of the past and move forward with a renewed sense of purpose and clarity. By embracing forgiveness as a path to inner peace, we can experience a profound transformation in our lives and relationships, leading to a greater sense of joy and fulfillment.

In the pursuit of eternal happiness, forgiveness is a crucial step towards healing past traumas and releasing emotional baggage that may be holding us back. By letting go of resentment and choosing to forgive, we can create a brighter future for ourselves and cultivate lasting joy and fulfillment in every moment. Embracing forgiveness as a path to inner peace is a powerful practice that can lead us towards a more fulfilling and meaningful life.

CHAPTER NINE

CONNECTING WITH NATURE AND THE OUTDOORS FOR
A SENSE OF PEACE AND HARMONY

"Connecting with Nature and the Outdoors for a Sense of Peace and Harmony" beckons us to rediscover the profound solace and beauty found in the natural world. This exploration celebrates the transformative power of immersing ourselves in the embrace of nature, where the cacophony of daily life gives way to tranquil serenity. Through mindful observation, outdoor adventures, and ecotherapy practices, it unveils the healing potential of communing with the earth. From awe-inspiring landscapes to the soothing rhythm of the wilderness, this narrative invites us to forge a deeper connection with nature, nurturing our spirits and fostering a profound sense of peace and harmony.

The benefits of spending time in nature for mental health

Spending time in nature has numerous benefits for our mental health and well-being. In today's fast-paced world, it's easy to get caught up in the hustle and bustle of daily life, leading to stress, anxiety, and feelings of overwhelm. However, by taking the time to connect with nature, we can find a sense of peace and tranquillity that can help to alleviate these negative emotions.

One of the key benefits of spending time in nature is the opportunity for mindfulness and meditation practices. Being in nature allows us to quiet our minds, focus on the present moment, and let go of worries and stress. By practicing mindfulness in nature, we can cultivate a sense of inner peace and contentment that can carry over into other areas of our lives.

In addition to mindfulness and meditation, spending time in nature can also help us cultivate gratitude and appreciation for the present moment. When we take the time to notice the beauty of the natural world around us – from the colours of a sunset to the sounds of a babbling brook – we can't help but feel a sense of awe and wonder. This appreciation for the present moment can lead to greater happiness and fulfillment in our lives.

Furthermore, connecting with nature can help us in our journey of self-discovery and personal growth. Nature has a way of reflecting back to us our own inner landscape, allowing us to gain insights into ourselves and our lives. Whether through a solitary hike in the woods or a quiet moment by the ocean, nature can provide the space and clarity we need to reflect on our goals, values, and desires.

Ultimately, spending time in nature can help us find a sense of peace and harmony in our lives. By immersing ourselves in the beauty and serenity of the natural world, we can reconnect with our true selves, find joy in the simple things, and experience a deeper sense of purpose and fulfillment. So, next time you're feeling overwhelmed or stressed, consider taking a walk in the woods, sitting by a lake, or simply gazing at the stars – you may just find the peace and happiness you've been searching for.

Engaging in outdoor activities for stress relief

Engaging in outdoor activities can be a powerful tool for reducing stress and finding peace in our fast-paced, modern world. Whether it's taking a leisurely walk in the park, hiking through a scenic trail, or simply sitting by a peaceful lake, connecting with nature can have a profound impact on our emotional well-being. For men and women seeking eternal happiness, spending time outdoors can provide a sense of tranquillity and harmony that is often hard to find in our daily lives.

Mindfulness and meditation practices are essential tools for finding peace and contentment in every moment. By immersing ourselves in the beauty of nature, we can cultivate a sense of mindfulness that allows us to fully appreciate the present moment. Whether it's feeling the warm sun on our skin, listening to the soothing sounds of birds chirping, or breathing in the fresh air, being outdoors can help us become more mindful and present in our daily lives.

Cultivating gratitude and appreciation for the present moment is another key aspect of finding happiness through outdoor activities. When we take the time to connect with nature and appreciate its beauty, we can develop a deeper sense of gratitude for the world around us. By focusing on the positive aspects of our surroundings, we can shift our perspective and find joy in even the simplest moments.

Finding happiness through self-discovery and personal growth is a journey that can be greatly enhanced by spending time in nature. The outdoors provides a space for reflection, introspection, and personal growth. Whether it's challenging ourselves with a new outdoor activity or simply taking a moment to appreciate the beauty of our surroundings, connecting with nature can help us discover more about ourselves and our place in the world.

Embracing simplicity and minimalism in our lives can lead to a more fulfilling and joyful existence. By spending time outdoors and connecting with the natural world, we can learn to appreciate the simple pleasures in life. Whether it's watching a sunset, feeling the wind on our face, or admiring the beauty of a flower, embracing simplicity can help us find lasting joy and fulfillment in every moment.

Finding peace and harmony through nature meditation

In the hustle and bustle of our modern lives, finding peace and harmony can feel like an elusive dream. However, one powerful way to connect with our inner selves and the world around us is through nature meditation. By immersing ourselves in the beauty and tranquillity of the natural world, we can cultivate a sense of calm and contentment that transcends the chaos of everyday life.

Nature meditation involves simply being present in nature, whether it's a walk in the woods, sitting by a babbling brook, or watching the sunset over the ocean. By focusing on the sights, sounds, and sensations of the natural world, we can quiet the chatter of our minds and tune into the peaceful energy that surrounds us. This practice can help us let go of stress, anxiety, and worries, allowing us to experience a profound sense of relaxation and well-being.

Through nature meditation, we can also deepen our connection to the earth and all living beings. By recognizing our interconnectedness with nature, we can cultivate a sense of gratitude and appreciation for the beauty and abundance that surrounds us. This awareness can inspire us to live more mindfully and sustainably, making choices that honour and protect the environment for future generations.

In addition to fostering peace and harmony within ourselves, nature meditation can also help us tap into a deeper sense of purpose and fulfillment. By aligning ourselves with the rhythms of the natural world, we can gain insight into our own inner workings and uncover our true desires and passions. This self-discovery can lead us on a path of personal growth and transformation, as we align our actions and intentions with our authentic selves.

Incorporating nature meditation into our daily lives can be a powerful tool for finding lasting joy and contentment. By taking the time to connect with the earth, we can nurture our spirits, heal past traumas, and release emotional baggage that may be holding us back. Through this practice, we can cultivate a sense of peace and harmony that extends beyond ourselves, creating a ripple effect of positivity and love in the world around us.

CHAPTER TEN

INCORPORATING SPIRITUAL PRACTICES AND BELIEFS INTO DAILY LIFE FOR A DEEPER SENSE OF PURPOSE AND FULFILLMENT

"Incorporating Spiritual Practices and Beliefs into Daily Life for a Deeper Sense of Purpose and Fulfillment" embarks on a journey of soulful exploration and awakening. This exploration celebrates the profound wisdom and guidance found in spiritual traditions, inviting individuals to weave these teachings into the fabric of their everyday existence. Through prayer, meditation, ritual, and mindful living, it unveils the transformative potential of aligning with a higher purpose. By nurturing a connection to the divine and honoring inner truths, this narrative offers a roadmap to fulfillment, guiding seekers towards a life imbued with meaning, compassion, and profound spiritual fulfillment.

Exploring different spiritual practices for inner peace

In the quest for eternal happiness, it is essential to explore different spiritual practices that can lead us to inner peace. These practices can vary greatly, from mindfulness and meditation techniques to cultivating gratitude and appreciation for the present moment. By delving into these practices, we can uncover a deeper sense of contentment and fulfillment in our lives.

Mindfulness and meditation practices are powerful tools for finding peace and contentment within ourselves. By focusing on the present moment and quieting the chatter of our minds, we can tap into a sense of inner calm and tranquillity. Through regular practice, we can learn to let go of negative thoughts and emotions, allowing us to experience a greater sense of peace and joy in our daily lives.

Cultivating gratitude and appreciation for the present moment is another essential practice for finding happiness. By taking the time to acknowledge and savour the blessings in our lives, we can shift our perspective from one of lack to one of abundance. This mindset shift can lead to a greater sense of contentment and fulfillment, as we learn to truly appreciate the beauty and joy that surrounds us.

Finding happiness through self-discovery and personal growth is also key to living a fulfilling life. By exploring our own values, beliefs, and desires, we can uncover our true purpose and passion in life. This journey of self-discovery can lead us to a deeper sense of fulfillment and joy, as we align our actions with our innermost desires and values.

Embracing simplicity and minimalism can also lead to a more fulfilling life. By decluttering our physical spaces and simplifying our lifestyles, we can create more room for joy, peace, and contentment. Letting go of material possessions and focusing on what truly brings us happiness can lead to a more meaningful and fulfilling life.

Connecting with your spiritual beliefs for guidance and support

Connecting with your spiritual beliefs can be a powerful source of guidance and support on your journey to eternal happiness. Whether you follow a specific religion or simply have a set of personal beliefs that resonate with you, tapping into your spiritual side can provide a sense of purpose and direction in life. By taking the time to explore and deepen your connection with your spiritual beliefs, you can find solace and comfort in times of uncertainty or difficulty.

Mindfulness and meditation practices can be particularly helpful in connecting with your spiritual beliefs. By quieting the mind and tuning into the present moment, you can create a space for spiritual insights and guidance to emerge. Whether you prefer to meditate in silence or incorporate prayer into your practice, taking the time to be still and listen to your inner voice can help you connect with a higher power or source of wisdom.

Cultivating gratitude and appreciation for the present moment is another important aspect of connecting with your spiritual beliefs. By focusing on the blessings and abundance in your life, you can shift your perspective from lack to abundance. This mindset of gratitude can help you feel more connected to the divine and foster a sense of peace and contentment in your daily life.

Finding happiness through self-discovery and personal growth is also essential in deepening your connection with your spiritual beliefs. By exploring your values, passions, and desires, you can align your life with your spiritual purpose and create a sense of fulfillment and meaning. Embracing simplicity and minimalism can also support your spiritual journey by helping you declutter your physical and mental space, allowing room for spiritual insights and growth.

Nurturing relationships and connections with are the key components of connecting with your spiritual beliefs. By fostering deep, meaningful connections with loved ones and like-minded individuals, you can create a supportive community that shares your values and beliefs. This sense of connection can bring joy and fulfillment into your life and help you feel supported on your spiritual path. By incorporating spiritual practices and beliefs into your daily life, you can cultivate a deeper sense of purpose and fulfillment, leading you on the joyful path to eternal happiness.

Living in alignment with your values for a fulfilling life

Living in alignment with your values is a key component of living a fulfilling life. When you are true to your values, you are living authentically and in harmony with your deepest beliefs and desires. This can lead to a sense of purpose and fulfillment that is unparalleled. In order to live in alignment with your values, it is important to first identify what those values are. Take some time to reflect on what is truly important to you and what you want your life to stand for.

Once you have identified your values, it is important to make choices and decisions that are in line with them. This may mean making sacrifices or saying no to things that do not align with your values. It may also mean standing up for what you believe in, even when it is difficult. Living in alignment with your values requires courage and conviction, but the rewards are well worth it.

One way to ensure that you are living in alignment with your values is to practice mindfulness and meditation. These practices can help you stay connected to your innermost self and make decisions from a place of clarity and awareness. By taking the time to quiet your mind and listen to your heart, you can ensure that you are acting in accordance with your values and not simply reacting to external pressures or influences.

Cultivating gratitude and appreciation for the present moment is another important aspect of living in alignment with your values. When you are grateful for what you have and appreciate the beauty of the world around you, you are more likely to make choices that are in line with your values. Gratitude can also help you stay focused on the positive aspects of your life, even in the face of challenges or obstacles.

Incorporating spiritual practices and beliefs into your daily life can also help you live in alignment with your values. Whether you follow a specific religion or simply have a personal set of beliefs, connecting with something greater than yourself can provide a sense of purpose and direction. By aligning your actions with your spiritual beliefs, you can live a life that is fulfilling and meaningful.

Embracing Eternal Happiness

As we reach the culmination of our journey along "The Joyful Path: A Guide to Eternal Happiness for Men and Women," it's essential to reflect on the transformative insights we've uncovered. Through the pages of this guide, we've explored the intricacies of happiness, delving deep into the essence of what it means to lead a truly fulfilling life.

In our pursuit of eternal happiness, we've discovered that joy isn't merely a destination but rather a continuous journey—an ongoing process of growth, self-discovery, and mindfulness. We've learned that happiness isn't found in external possessions or fleeting pleasures but resides within the depths of our souls, waiting to be awakened and nurtured.

Throughout this book, we've explored various principles and practices that can guide us toward a life of enduring joy. From cultivating gratitude and embracing simplicity to fostering meaningful connections and nurturing our inner peace, each chapter has offered invaluable insights and practical tools for living a more fulfilling existence.

As we bid farewell to these pages, let us remember that the journey doesn't end here. Instead, let it serve as a springboard for our ongoing quest for happiness and fulfillment. Let us continue to walk the joyful path with courage, compassion, and an unwavering commitment to living our best lives.

In closing, I invite you to carry the wisdom of "The Joyful Path" with you as you navigate the ups and downs of life's ever-unfolding journey. May its teachings inspire you; its lessons empower you, and its message resonate deeply within your heart.

With heartfelt gratitude and boundless optimism, may we embark on the next chapter of our lives with renewed purpose and a steadfast dedication to embracing eternal happiness.

Wishing you joy, peace, and abundance on your joyful path.

Appendix

Here's a diverse list of further readings that touch upon themes of joy, happiness, and spiritual fulfillment:

1. "The Art of Happiness" by Dalai Lama and Howard Cutler - Explores the Dalai Lama's teachings on finding joy and contentment.

2. "The Power of Now" by Eckhart Tolle - Offers insights on living in the present moment to attain inner peace and happiness.

3. "The Happiness Project" by Gretchen Rubin - Chronicles one woman's year-long journey to increase her happiness and fulfillment.

4. "Man's Search for Meaning" by Viktor E. Frankl - Reflects on finding purpose and meaning in life, even in the face of suffering.

5. "The Alchemist" by Paulo Coelho - A fable about following one's dreams and finding fulfillment on life's journey.

6. "The Joy of Living: Unlocking the Secret and Science of Happiness" by Yongey Mingyur Rinpoche - Combines Tibetan Buddhism with modern science to explore happiness.

7. "The Four Agreements" by Don Miguel Ruiz - Offers practical wisdom for personal freedom and happiness based on ancient Toltec teachings.

8. "Siddhartha" by Hermann Hesse - Follows the journey of Siddhartha as he seeks enlightenment and happiness.

9. "The Little Book of Hygge: Danish Secrets to Happy Living" by Meik Wiking - Explores the Danish concept of hygge, focusing on coziness and contentment.

10. "The Book of Joy: Lasting Happiness in a Changing World" by Dalai Lama, Desmond Tutu, and Douglas Abrams - Shares insights from a week-long conversation between the Dalai Lama and Desmond Tutu on finding joy in difficult times.

These books offer a variety of perspectives and insights into the pursuit of happiness and fulfillment, each with its own valuable lessons to impart.

Epilogue

As the journey along The Joyful Path draws to a close, its teachings continue to resonate deeply within the hearts of men and women alike. Each reader, enriched by the wisdom found within its pages, now carries a radiant light of joy and fulfillment.

Through the trials faced and triumphs celebrated, the lessons learned have become the foundation upon which they build their lives. United in purpose and spirit, they walk confidently towards a future illuminated by eternal happiness.

Yet, the true essence of The Joyful Path lies not only in its guidance but in the connections forged along the way. Communities thrive, bound by a shared commitment to love, compassion, and understanding.

And so, as the sun sets on this chapter, a new dawn awaits. With hearts overflowing with gratitude, men and women step forward, emboldened by the enduring promise of joy found within The Joyful Path.

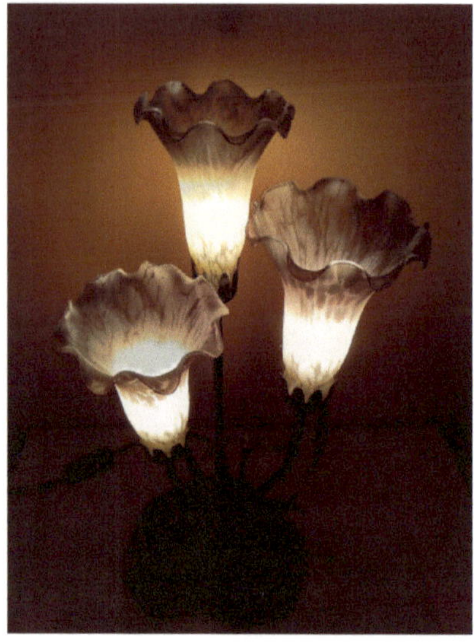

"Let there be light, peace and happiness in the hearts of all beings"

ABOUT THE AUTHOR

In the bustling rhythm of the workday, Prajaspri finds purpose and fulfillment, dedicating to a career path rich with challenges and growth. Yet, beyond the confines of professional life, lies a colourful tapestry of passions waiting to unfold. A culinary enthusiast at heart, Prajaspri channels creativity and love into the kitchen, where flavours blend and memories are shared with cherished family and friends. Alongside this, Prajaspri finds solace in the gentle verses of poetry, weaving emotions into words, and expressing the depth of the soul. Though the world's vast landscapes remain largely unexplored, Prajaspri dreams of future adventures, eager to immerse themselves in new cultures and experiences, each promising to enrich life with stories untold and horizons yet unseen. With a thirst for knowledge and a passion for well-being, Prajaspri advocates for a lifestyle grounded in health, balance, and stress-free living. Through the medium of writing, including poetry, Prajaspri shares insights and inspirations, inviting others to join in the journey towards a brighter, more fulfilling existence.